The Menopause Advice:

Take Charge of Your Health through Feminism and Science.

Dr. Olivia Williams.

AUTHOR'S NOTE:
The information provided in this book on menopause is for educational and informational purposes only. It is not intended to be a substitute for professional medical advice, diagnosis, or treatment. Always seek the advice of your physician or other qualified healthcare provider with any questions you may have regarding a medical condition.

Table of Contents

INTRODUCTION

The life of a human female is marked from adolescent years by monthly menstruation which terminates commonly between the age of 40 and 60 years. This stage is termed as "Menopause". The name "menopause" originates from the Greek word "month" and "cessation", alluding to the final menstrual cycle. A transition phase in mid-life, spanning 2 to 10 years, when menstruation is less regular is called *Perimenopause.* The transition phase preceding menopause is sometimes referred to as *Perimenopause.* During this transition stage before menopause, the production of mature eggs in a woman's ovaries reduces and ovulation becomes irregular. At the same time, the synthesis of estrogen and progesterone diminishes. It is the substantial reduction in estrogen levels that produces most of the symptoms of menopause. Menopause is a normal physiological and natural process. The World Health Organization (WHO) defines *Menopause* as the permanent cessation of menstruation owing to loss of ovarian follicular activity at the end of reproductive life. Before a woman enters Menopause, she goes through Perimenopause which normally occurs in a woman's late 30s or early 40s but can start earlier or later for certain women. During perimenopause, hormone levels, particularly estrogen, vary, which can produce a range of symptoms. *Menopause* is the era of a woman's life when menstrual cycles end. It affects all women as they mature. The symptoms of menopause are caused by hormone insufficiency (estrogen and progesterone), which happens when periods stop, often between the ages of 45 and 55; the average age of menopause is 51. It is impacted by both hereditary and environmental factors. Due to the increased life expectancy of women, postmenopausal years cover more than one-third of the entire female life span.

Common symptoms of perimenopause include irregular periods, hot flashes, night sweats, mood swings, sleep difficulties, vaginal dryness, reduced libido, and changes in skin and hair texture. These symptoms might vary in strength and length and can have a substantial influence on a woman's quality of life. Perimenopause can continue anywhere from a few months to several years and ends when a woman has not had a menstrual cycle for 12 consecutive months. It is crucial for women to talk to their healthcare practitioner about their symptoms and management choices, which may include lifestyle modifications, hormone therapy, or other drugs.

Though natural events of estrogen deficiency of menopause herald a variety of potential problems that can affect the quality of life, specific concerns include subjective symptoms such as vasomotor instability, i.e., hot flushes, psychological and psychomotor disorders, menstrual irregularities, vaginal dryness, genitourinary dysfunction, and osteoporosis which have implications for long-term health.

So, doctors and menopausal women are both interested in and deserve knowledge of the symptoms and the foundation for treatment prescription targeted at easing symptoms and lowering eventual health risks.

Natural menopause is regarded to have happened after 12 consecutive months of amenorrhea, for which there is no other clear medical or physiological explanation. When a woman gets no menstrual flow following perimenopause for 12 consecutive months, it is believed that she has entered her menopausal period.

Post-menopause is the period of time after a woman has gone 12 straight months without a monthly cycle. It signals the conclusion of the menopausal transition and the commencement of the post-reproductive period of a woman's life. During post-menopause, the body continues to adjust to the reduced levels of estrogen, progesterone, and other hormones that occur after menopause. Women may endure certain persistent symptoms from perimenopause, such as hot flashes, vaginal dryness, and mood disturbances, although these symptoms normally get less severe with time. Women in post-menopause are also at an elevated risk for certain health issues, such as osteoporosis, heart disease, and some malignancies.

It is vital for women to maintain a healthy lifestyle, including regular exercise and a balanced diet, and to undertake recommended health tests to control these risks. Hormone replacement therapy (HRT) is occasionally used to control symptoms and minimize health risks in postmenopausal women, but it is not suited for everyone and should be carefully examined in collaboration with a healthcare practitioner. Menopause occurs with the final menstrual cycle, which is recognized with certainty only in hindsight a year or more after the event. A suitable independent biological marker for the occurrence does not exist.

When a woman undergoes a menstrual transition, her estrogen and other hormone levels change as she ages, there is also a decline in the ovaries, reproduction ability reduces, etc., and the body generally begins to transform. At this stage, the menstrual cycle is frequently more unpredictable.

The graphic below demonstrates this change.

Stages of Ovarian Function in a Woman's Cycle.

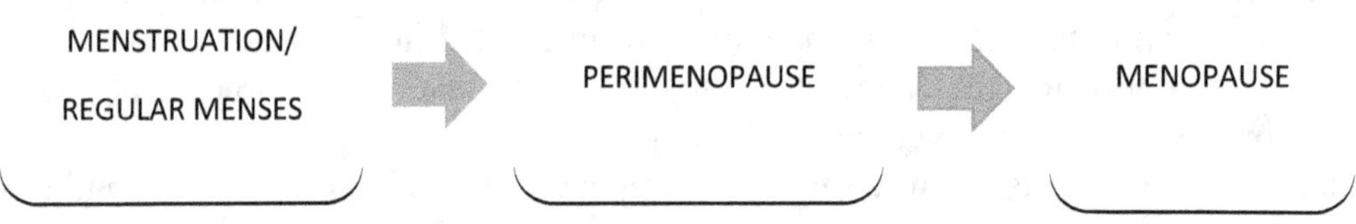

Menopause is marked by hormonal changes that can affect physical, emotional, and psychological well-being. Despite its prevalence, it remains a topic that is often misunderstood, and many women are left feeling uncertain and anxious about what to expect. In this book, we aim to provide a comprehensive guide to menopause, exploring its biology, symptoms, and effects on women's health and quality of life. We will also delve into the cultural and societal attitudes surrounding menopause, as well as the various treatments and strategies available to manage its effects. Whether you are experiencing menopause yourself or seeking to support someone who is, this book will offer valuable insights and practical advice to navigate this important life transition.

CHAPTER 1

Is Menopause a stage to be considered significant in a Woman's cycle?

Yes, menopause is an important period in a woman's life cycle, as it signifies the end of reproductive years and the commencement of a new era of life. Menopause is a normal biological process that happens in all women as they age, often in their late 40s or early 50s, and can continue for many years. In addition to the physical symptoms, menopause can also have emotional and social effects. It may be a period of contemplation and transition for women, as they adjust to changes in their bodies and their responsibilities in society.

Some women may endure thoughts of loss or grief, while others may welcome this new chapter of life with a sense of emancipation and empowerment. In addition to the physical symptoms, menopause can also have emotional and social effects. Some women may endure thoughts of loss or grief, while others may welcome this new chapter of life with a sense of emancipation and empowerment. It may be a period of contemplation and transition for women, as they adjust to changes in their bodies and their responsibilities in society. We can do better by embracing the concept of a feminist menopause. Women ought to experience these changes in their bodies prepared with knowledge and free of fear, shame, or concealment.

In certain communities, a woman's worth is related to her ovarian function, and the end of her reproductive life marks the end of her productive life. The medical profession should offer women significantly more knowledge about how their hormones, alter in midlife and what they should expect, and what may be handled with medical treatment. The implications of Menopause may be psychological, health and physical, emotional, and social, or could possibly affect your working life.

The subsequent paragraphs explain how great they impact the menopausal woman.

Health and Physical consequences

1. Hot flashes and nocturnal sweats: These are the most frequent symptoms of menopause and can create rapid feelings of warmth or heat that spread throughout the body, sometimes accompanied by perspiration and chills.

2. Vaginal and urinary alterations: Decreased estrogen levels can induce changes in vaginal and urinary function, including vaginal dryness, itching, and discomfort during intercourse, as well as urinary incontinence and increased frequency of urinary tract infections.

3. Bone loss and higher risk of fractures: Decreased estrogen levels can lead to bone loss and an increased risk of fractures, particularly in the hips, spine, and wrists.

4. Changes in skin and hair: Decreased estrogen levels can also cause changes in skin and hair, including dryness, thinning, and loss of suppleness.

5. Sleep difficulties: Hot flashes and night sweats can induce sleep disruptions, and menopause can also be related with other sleep disorders such as insomnia and sleep apnea.

6. Weight increase: Some women may suffer weight gain or changes in body composition after menopause, which can be connected to hormonal changes, age, and lifestyle factors.

7. cardiovascular disease risk: After menopause, women have an increased risk of getting cardiovascular disease, which is considered to be connected to changes in estrogen levels.

8. Sexual function: Menopause can also influence sexual function, including reduced desire, vaginal dryness, and pain during intercourse.

These physical consequences of menopause can have a substantial influence on a woman's quality of life.

Emotional and Social Implications.

Menopause is to be expected as a woman ages but it occurs to some women as a surprise thus, they find it tough to embrace the changes and symptoms that accompany it. Some of the most prevalent social effects of menopause include:

1. events in family dynamics: Menopause typically corresponds with other life events, such as children leaving home, which can disrupt family dynamics and relationships.

2. Changes in social roles: Menopause can also be accompanied by changes in social duties and obligations, such as retirement or caregiving for aged parents or grandkids.

3. Stigma and stereotypes: Menopause has historically been stigmatized and stereotyped as a negative or disruptive condition, which can damage a woman's self-esteem and social relationships.

4. Impact on sexuality and intimacy: Menopause can also have repercussions for sexual function and intimacy, which can damage a woman's relationships and

Low self-esteem, lack of confidence, low mood and feelings of melancholy or despair, poor focus, commonly characterized as 'brain fog', forgotten words, and worry are prevalent emotions at this stage. This can be due to the reduction in estrogen levels but in certain undeveloped nations, certain symptoms like hot flashes are connected with witchcraft, where these women are neglected by family and society and transported to witches' camps with little or no care.

The stress of not being able to live their best lives or amass wealth before midlife, when they can work sporadically or leave their jobs, affects other women. They load themselves with these and finally grow melancholy.

Psychological Implications

Menopause can have a number of psychological ramifications for women, as they adjust to changes in their bodies and their responsibilities in society. Some of the frequent psychological effects of menopause include:

1. Mood changes: Fluctuating hormone levels during menopause can produce mood swings, irritability, and sadness in some women.

2. Anxiety: Some women may have anxiety or panic episodes during menopause, which can be connected to hormonal changes, as well as other variables such as stress and lifestyle changes.

3. Loss of identity: For some women, menopause can be a period of introspection and transition, as they adjust to changes in their bodies and their responsibilities in society. This might lead to emotions of loss or uncertainty about their identity and purpose.

4. Decreased self-esteem: Changes in physical appearance, such as weight gain or changes in skin and hair texture, can significantly impair a woman's self-esteem and body image during menopause.

5. Sexual function: Menopause can also influence sexual function, including reduced desire, vaginal dryness, and pain during intercourse. This might have psychological ramifications for women since it can influence their self-image and relationships.

It is crucial for women to talk to their healthcare practitioner about any psychological symptoms they may be having during menopause, since there are a number of management options available, including counseling, medication, and lifestyle modifications. Women can also benefit from support and knowledge about menopause, and connecting with other women who are going through the same experience can be beneficial in handling the psychological consequences of menopause.

Working life.

Menopause can influence the professional lives of women in a number of ways. Some women may develop physical symptoms, such as hot flashes and night sweats, which can be disruptive to work and limit their ability to focus and do everyday chores. Other women may have psychological symptoms, such as mood fluctuations and anxiety, which can compromise their general well-being and job performance.

Menopause can also have repercussions for women's career trajectories, as it frequently happens during a period when women are at the top of their careers. Women may need to take time from work to manage symptoms or attend medical appointments, which can hinder their productivity and career growth. Women may also encounter prejudice or bias in the job based on age or views of menopause as a bad or disruptive condition.

However, menopause may also be a period of empowerment and rejuvenation for women, as they reflect on their beliefs and priorities and make adjustments to enhance their general well-being. Some women may want to take on new challenges or explore new career paths at this time, and companies may encourage this by offering flexible work arrangements, education and resources on menopause, and a culture of inclusion and support for women of all ages and life stages.

Job discrimination: Some women may encounter discrimination or bias in the workplace based on beliefs of menopause as a bad or disruptive condition. In most organizations, workers are expected to retire at age 60 and some employees are ready to employ women over age 45 because they will soon approach menopause and are thought to be less productive. Overall, menopause can have complicated ramifications for women's work lives, and it is crucial for employers and colleagues to help women during this time and build a work environment that is inclusive and supportive of women of all ages and life stages.

Overall, menopause is a key period in a woman's life cycle, and it is vital for women to take care of their physical and mental health at this time. Women should communicate with their healthcare professionals about their symptoms and management choices, and maintain a healthy lifestyle to promote their general well-being.

CHAPTER 2
The Biological Breakdown of Menopause.

Most typically, the "biology of menopause" is linked with "the biomedical model of menopause." The biomedical approach highlights the key relevance of estrogen and has an overwhelming focus on illness. A more comprehensive biological paradigm is put forth that emphasizes the significance of hormones in healthy functioning. Hormones are team players in complicated, multidetermined systems that have a function. Hormones function in combination with other physiological systems and with sensory and social inputs. Human biology is both similar to and different from that of other species. The consequences of these assumptions for understanding menopause are examined, notably the sorts of questions that are asked and the kinds of data needed before judgments are formed in relation to clinically significant regions. A more comprehensive biological model of menopause offers a context within which health-related issues can be viewed from an angle that is both more sensitive to individual differences and more holistic in nature.

Actually, menopause is a hormonal change that occurs as one biological stage of life ends and another begins, similar to the puberty transition. Menopause is a result of changes in both the ovaries and the brain. Women are born with a finite number of eggs, or oocytes, and decades of ovulation lead the supply and quality of oocytes to diminish, altering the generation of estrogens and progestogens as well as the brain's sensitivity to these hormones. Oocytes, commonly known as egg cells or ova, are female reproductive cells or gametes that are generated in the ovaries. Oocytes are among the largest cells in the human body that can be seen with the unaided eye. They are also essential for reproduction. During ovulation, one or more mature oocytes are released from the ovaries and move via the fallopian tubes, where they may be fertilized by sperm and grow into an embryo. If fertilization does not occur, the egg is lost along with the uterine lining during menstruation. Oocytes contain half of the genetic material needed to generate a new human being, and faults or anomalies in oocyte development can lead to infertility or genetic diseases.

Eventually, a woman gets her last menstrual cycle—an occurrence that's usually regarded as the hallmark of menopause. However, the process as a whole doesn't really involve the event that much. The final menstrual cycle might be significant for understanding when to discontinue contraception, and its arrival can impact how

physicians analyze irregular menstrual flow. But what actually matters for the day-to-day lives of individuals with ovaries starts years before the final menstrual cycle and lasts a lifetime, since the hormonal changes of the transitions might raise the risk of ailments such as heart disease, osteoporosis, stroke, dementia, etc. But since many women are unaware of the basic biology of menopause, they are unsure of what to expect when their regular menstrual cycles stop. They may worry that a hot-flush inferno would leave them drenched with perspiration at work, or dread confronting the issue of vaginal dryness with their sexual partner. Therefore, it is important to understand the biology of menopause for the benefit of all women as well as for the study of gynecology and feminine health.

Age-related alterations occur throughout the reproductive lives of typical healthy women. From the age of 20, the menstrual interval steadily shortens and becomes increasingly regular until perimenopause. This is connected to a shortening of the follicular phase rather than the luteal phase of the cycle. The follicular phase is the first phase of the menstrual cycle, which begins on the first day of menstruation and concludes with ovulation. During this period, the body prepares for future pregnancy by forming and maturing a follicle in one of the ovaries, which houses an egg.

The follicular phase is governed by hormones, notably follicle-stimulating hormone (FSH), which encourages the formation and development of follicles in the ovaries. As the follicles expand, they release estrogen, which thickens the uterine lining in preparation for pregnancy.

Typically, the follicular period lasts 10 to 14 days, though this can vary from person to person. Ovulation happens when the dominant follicle ruptures and releases the developed egg into the fallopian tube, where it may be fertilized by sperm. The luteal phase is the second phase of the menstrual cycle, which follows ovulation and concludes with the onset of the next menstruation. During this phase, the body prepares for prospective pregnancy by releasing high amounts of progesterone to maintain the thicker uterine lining that was grown up during the follicular phase.

The luteal phase is governed by hormones, particularly luteinizing hormone (LH) and progesterone.

After ovulation, the remaining follicle in the ovary converts into the corpus luteum, which releases progesterone to prepare the uterus for the implantation of a fertilized egg. If fertilization does not occur, the corpus luteum degenerates, progesterone levels decline, and the uterus loses its lining, culminating in menstruation. The duration of the luteal phase can vary from person to person, but it typically lasts 10 to 14 days. It is frequently thought to have a more consistent duration than the follicular phase. Hormonal abnormalities during the luteal phase can contribute to different menstrual illnesses, such as irregular cycles, premenstrual syndrome (PMS), and infertility.

Thus, the potential for reproduction falls and disappears when the ovaries become deprived of follicles. Serum follicle-stimulating hormone (FSH) concentration is enhanced during the follicular phase in older women who are still menstruating regularly, but serum inhibin levels are lowered in both the follicular and luteal phases. The key factor determining the shift from normal menses to perimenopause and subsequent menopause appears to be the amount of the remnant primordial follicle pool. Menopause is also linked with a large reduction in plasma concentrations of sex hormones, a rise in the concentrations of gonadotrophins, and alterations in other hormones such as inhibin.

The link between FSH secretion, ageing and feedback inhibition by estradiol, inhibin, or other now unmeasured variables in women with regular menses, has to be explained. At age 29, fecundability starts to decline. Fecundability refers to the possibility of achieving a pregnancy in one menstrual cycle or one month of unprotected sexual intercourse. It is affected by a number of factors, including aging, hormonal imbalances, lifestyle choices, and underlying medical conditions. Fecundability may be measured by the time it takes for a couple to conceive after they start attempting to conceive. For instance, a couple's fecundability is higher when they get pregnant after just one month of trying, whereas it is lower when it takes them more than a year to do so.

Knowing the factors that impact fecundability can help people and couples make educated decisions about their reproductive health and boost their chances of conceiving. Some measures to promote fecundability include keeping a healthy weight, lowering stress, quitting smoking, limiting alcohol intake, and tracking ovulation to optimize the timing of sexual intercourse.

The oocytes and endometrium play vital roles in fertilization and early pregnancy, yet the quality of these is influenced by age. Oocytes are produced from the ovaries during ovulation and move into the fallopian tubes, where they may be fertilized by sperm. The quality of the oocyte can determine whether fertilization happens, since older or defective Oocytes may be less likely to be fertilized or may lead to chromosomal abnormalities in the developing embryo.

Once fertilization occurs, the growing embryo passes through the fallopian tubes and implants into the endometrium of the uterus. The thickness and quality of the endometrium play a key role in early pregnancy success and successful implantation. The endometrium must be thick enough to enable implantation and give nutrition to the growing fetus. It must also be receptive to hormonal cues and have enough blood supply to support the developing embryo.

If there are concerns with the quality of the oocyte or the thickness and quality of the endometrium, fertilization and implantation may be less likely to occur or may result in early pregnancy loss. This may be a factor in infertility or recurrent miscarriages.

Before a woman is born, oocytes are produced in her ovaries, and as she gets older, fewer oocytes are produced. By the time a woman reaches her late 30s and 40s, the quality and number of her remaining oocytes may diminish, which can make it more difficult to conceive and raise the chance of genetic abnormalities in kids. The endometrium is also impacted by ageing, since the periodic changes it experiences during the menstrual cycle become less predictable and less receptive to hormonal cues. This can lead to irregular periods, severe bleeding, and an increased risk of illnesses such as endometrial hyperplasia and cancer.

Additionally, the thickness and quality of the endometrium may deteriorate with age, which can make it more difficult for a fertilized egg to implant and raise the risk of pregnancy difficulties. Overall, while both oocytes and the endometrium are impacted by age, the loss in oocyte quality and quantity is typically thought to have a bigger influence on female fertility and reproductive health.

The endometrium is the inner lining of the uterus, which is the female reproductive organ where a fertilized egg implants and matures throughout pregnancy.

The endometrium is a complex and dynamic tissue that undergoes cyclic changes throughout the menstrual cycle in response to hormonal cues. The endometrium is lost during menstruation if a fertilized egg does not implant, and the cycle starts over.

The thickness and shape of the endometrium are essential determinants of female fertility and can be influenced by many medical problems, including polyps, fibroids, and endometriosis.

Menopause is a stage of life when the ovaries are devoid of oocytes, and the cyclical activity of gonadotrophins, peptides, and steroids is lost. At the end of the final menses, only a few follicles remain. There are no endocrine indicators that signify the last cycle. Hence, menopause can only be detected retroactively when there are no additional menses. The chance of being menopausal increases with the length of amenorrhea and age. Considerable evidence demonstrates that both blood FSH and serum inhibin are indicators of the number and/or quality of follicles remaining in the ovary. There is also evidence that the age of menopause, itself, is a significant indicator of the general ageing status of the individual.

CHAPTER 3
Can Menopause be a Positive Experience?

Yes, menopause may be a wonderful experience for many women. While menopause is generally linked with physical, emotional, and psychological problems, it may also be a period of development, self-reflection, and empowerment.

One of the good elements of menopause is that it signifies the end of a woman's reproductive phase, which can bring a sense of relief or liberation. Women who have gone through menopause may no longer have to worry about pregnancy or birth control, which might allow them to focus on other elements of their lives, such as their work, hobbies, or personal growth.

Moreover, menopause can also give a chance for women to emphasize their own needs and interests. During their reproductive years, women typically have to juggle the pressures of parenting, career, and other commitments. However, menopause may be a period when women can focus on themselves and their aspirations, which can be empowering.

In addition, menopause may also be a time of self-discovery and personal growth. Women who have gone through menopause may have earned tremendous life experience and insight, which may assist their families, communities, and workplaces. They may also have more time and energy to explore new interests or hobbies, which may be enlightening and gratifying.

Furthermore, menopause may also be a period of greater closeness and connection with partners. While women may suffer changes in their sexual desire or sexual function following menopause, they may also have more time and emotional energy to dedicate to their relationships. Moreover, women who have gone through menopause may no longer have to worry about the chance of pregnancy, which might allow them to enjoy sexual activity more freely.

The transition to menopause may also be a period of contemplation and inspiration. Although changes of any type can be fundamentally painful, many women find a sense of freedom and expect personal improvement. Menopause is a crossroads, a moment to renew yourself, adjust your emphasis and start exploring your own needs more. It is an opportunity to return to your aspirations, revitalize a rusty job or establish a new one, focus on your health and wellness, go on a pilgrimage, travel … anything your heart wishes. Some noteworthy favorable implications of Menopause are:

Say goodbye to Menstrual Flow

Menopause signifies the end of the monthly cycle, which for many women is a reason for joy in itself. It means no more fiddling with tampons or pads, no more fear about leaking, and no more period cramps. And after the perimenopausal years, when periods typically become erratic and bleeding may be severe, it puts an end to the guessing game of when your period is going to start or cease. Some women are even constrained to their houses on days when bleeding is heavy, for them, menopause may be extremely freeing.

End of Premenstrual Syndrome (PMS)

In the week or two before your period, premenstrual syndrome (PMS) can induce several physical and emotional symptoms, ranging from breast soreness and headache pain to food cravings and irritability. PMS is highly common. In perimenopause, PMS can temporarily worsen as estrogen levels rise and fall. All the better, therefore, to have PMS disappear after menopause.

Enjoy Sex without Worrying about Pregnancy

Women in menopause can enjoy sex without having to fret about a possible pregnancy. For some women of different ethnic groups, sex without thinking about pregnancy is frequently cited as one of the benefits of menopause. After discovering that you no longer have to worry about the unplanned consequence of sex, you may enjoy it more once you enter menopause.

No Hormonal Headaches

Certain scientific findings reveal that women are impacted by headaches three times more commonly than males. According to research, about 70 percent of these women get menstrual migraines, headaches that correlate with ovulation and menstruation. Like other migraines, these headaches involve throbbing pain on one side of the head, occasionally accompanied by nausea, vomiting, and light- or sound-sensitivity. In a normal monthly cycle, changing amounts of the hormones estrogen and progesterone can produce menstrual migraines. But after menopause, levels of estrogen and progesterone reduce, and frequently the number of hormonal headaches declines too.

Shrinkage of Uterine Fibroids

Many women entering their 50s acquire fibroids, uterine tumors that are nearly often benign. Fibroids grow when estrogen levels in the body are high – during pregnancy when levels of estrogen and progesterone increase, and in perimenopause when estrogen levels can range from low to high. If fibroid symptoms, including discomfort, heavy menstrual blood, and strain on the bladder are severe, doctors may

consider surgery. Fortunately, fibroids generally cease growing or shrink when women reach menopause and estrogen levels fall. For women who have been charting fibroid growth hoping to avoid surgery, or for those who have heavy periods due to fibroids, menopause is welcome.

An opportunity to Take Stock

Menopause is a natural time for women to take stock of their lives. Many opt to take a new look at their relationships, their careers, the methods they're caring for their health, and the ways they wish to use their energy. It's important to take advantage of this wakeup call and put your best foot forward as you move along. You can ask yourself if you are moving in the direction you want to go, both professionally and emotionally, and whether the manner you are spending your time is meaningful to you.

Greater Self-Assurance

It is not rare for postmenopausal women to report feeling powerful, partly because of the physiologic changes that take place in menopause and partly because of the time in life at which menopause occurs. Women are often relieved not to have monthly periods with the accompanying risk of pregnancy, mood swings, and other PMS symptoms. Your children are growing older and you are freed to pursue your professional and personal ambitions at the same time. After 50-plus years of life experience, including the ups and downs of relationships, child-rearing, and careers, women are more likely to go after what they want with a greater sense of confidence that they can handle whatever comes their way.

A Time to Take Risks

After menopause, you have a third of your life to live, you may still take initiatives and new ideas without holding back. This is a message that women in menopause are eager to hear because midlife is the time when women are prone to take greater chances. Some move occupations, possibly converting a passion into a company. Others attempt online dating or other daring pastimes like mountain climbing or figure skating. If there's something you've been putting on wait, there's no time like the present to sample what life has to offer.

Focus on Caring for Yourself
With children grown or on their way to independence and a profession that's well established, women in menopause have more time to take care of themselves. Many women in menopause are receptive to making changes that will maintain or improve their health. These changes can start with receiving frequent health check-ups and routine health screenings, such as mammograms and Pap tests. You can also put your best foot forward by eating a nutritious diet that's low in fat and high in fruits and vegetables, and by obtaining regular physical activity - everything from walking and bicycling to gardening and housekeeping counts. It is also crucial to take time out and relieve stress; practices such as meditation, relaxation techniques, or tai chi can assist.

Connecting With Other Menopausal Women
When heat flashes have you peeling off layers of clothes or when you can't remember what that one thing was that you came to the store for, you're likely to sense a kinship with any woman as sweaty or forgetful as yourself. Talking — and frequently laughing — with other women about the menopausal symptoms you're experiencing may be beneficial by comforting you that you're not alone. Not only do women offer coping tactics and sympathy and understanding, but sharing their tales gives them strength to face the world, knowing that they're in good company.
Menopause may be a wonderful experience for many people. While it may come with obstacles, such as physical ailments or emotional shifts, it may also be a period of development, empowerment, and self-discovery. Women who have gone through menopause should be acknowledged for their fortitude, adaptation, and the tremendous contributions they continue to make to their families, communities, and workplaces.

CHAPTER 4
Is Early Menopause Normal? Why does it occur?

Early menopause, also known as premature menopause, is when a woman enters menopause before the age of 40. This can develop spontaneously, owing to some reasons, or as a result of medical procedures, such as surgery or chemotherapy. The most prevalent cause of early menopause is premature ovarian failure, which happens when the ovaries stop working normally and no longer generate enough estrogen and other hormones. This can happen for a variety of causes, including heredity, autoimmune illnesses, radiation or chemotherapy, and some medical therapies. Women who experience early menopause may have symptoms comparable to those of women going through natural menopause, such as hot flashes, nocturnal sweats, vaginal dryness, mood swings, and reduced libido. They are also at an elevated risk for certain health disorders, including osteoporosis, heart disease, and depression. Early menopause can have a severe influence on a woman's fertility, since she may no longer be able to conceive naturally.

Causes of Premature Menopause
The following are some of the reasons of early or premature menopause:
1. Natural decline in reproductive hormones. As you enter your late 30s, your ovaries begin to produce less estrogen and progesterone, the chemicals that govern menstruation, and your fertility begins to diminish.
Menstrual cycles in your 40s may be brown. Women who experience premature or early menopause have lower estrogen levels, which raises their long-term risk of osteoporosis and heart disease. Menopause can be caused by anything that destroys your ovaries or prevents your body from producing estrogen. Many of the symptoms of early menopause are similar to those of premature menopause, as periods lengthen or shorten, get heavier or lighter, and become more or less regular. Eventually, by age 51 on average, your ovaries stop producing eggs and you stop having periods.
2. Oophorectomy (removal of the ovaries). Your ovaries create hormones that govern the menstrual cycle, such as estrogen and progesterone. Menopause occurs immediately after surgery to remove your ovaries. Your periods stop, and hot flashes and other menopausal symptoms are more likely to strike. Because hormonal changes occur quickly rather than gradually over time, the signs and symptoms might be severe.

3. Hysterectomy (removal of the uterus but not the ovaries) does not generally result in quick menopause. Even if you no longer have periods, your ovaries continue to generate eggs as well as estrogen and progesterone.

Chemotherapy and radiation treatment are two options. These cancer treatments can cause menopause, resulting in symptoms such as hot flashes during or immediately after treatment. Because the cessation of menstruation (and fertility) is not necessarily permanent after chemotherapy, birth control techniques may still be required. Radiation treatment only affects ovarian function when it is focused on the ovaries. Other regions of the body, such as breast tissue or the head and neck, will not be affected by radiation therapy.

5. Ovarian insufficiency, primary. Premature menopause affects about 1% of women before the age of 40. Premature menopause can be caused by your ovaries' inability to generate normal amounts of reproductive hormones (primary ovarian insufficiency), which can be caused by hereditary causes or an autoimmune condition. However, in many cases, no reason of early menopause can be identified. Hormone treatment is often suggested for these women until the natural age of menopause to safeguard the brain, heart, and bones.

Other risk factors include a family history of early menopause, having your first period before the age of 11, chromosomal abnormalities such as Fragile X or Turner's syndrome, autoimmune diseases such as rheumatoid arthritis, Crohn's disease, or thyroid disease, smoking, myalgia encephalomyelitis/chronic fatigue syndrome (ME/CFS), having HIV or AIDS, and infections such as mumps.

Premature or early menopause can have unknown causes. This is true for up to 50% of the population. Women who undergo early menopause may investigate alternate choices, such as egg donation or adoption if they desire to have children.

It is crucial for women who experience early menopause to talk to their healthcare practitioner about their choices for managing symptoms and minimizing their risk of health issues. Hormone replacement therapy (HRT) is widely used to control symptoms and minimize the risk of osteoporosis, but it is not suited for everyone and should be carefully explored in collaboration with a healthcare practitioner.

Apart from the scientific basis behind this, inherited factors might cause this to happen. Similar to how early menstruation occurs in some families, some women may also experience early menopause. It is still advisable to consult your gynecologist for diagnosis and treatment.

CHAPTER 5

The Metamorphosis of Menopause; Strength, Size, and Shape Changes.

Menopause metamorphosis refers to the physical, mental, and hormonal changes that women go through as they approach menopause. A woman's ovaries stop producing eggs and produce less estrogen and progesterone during menopause. This might result in a number of symptoms, such as hot flashes, night sweats, vaginal dryness, mood swings, and sleep difficulties. Menopause symptoms can vary from woman to woman, with some suffering few or no symptoms and others experiencing more severe symptoms that might interfere with everyday living. The menopausal transition can potentially last several years, with some women having symptoms for several years before and following menopause.

While the menopausal transition might be difficult, it is vital to remember that it is a natural and typical phase of life.

Many women in their forties and fifties make the shift from a pear-shaped figure (wide hips and thighs with more weight below the waist) to an apple-shaped body (broad waist and belly with more weight above the waist).

Menopause can affect a woman's strength in numerous ways:

1. Hormonal changes: The synthesis of estrogen and progesterone decreases after menopause, which can contribute to a loss of muscle mass and strength.

2. Physical changes: Menopause is also connected with changes in body composition, such as an increase in body fat and a decrease in muscular mass, which can result in a loss of strength. Reduced physical activity: Because of symptoms such as hot flashes, sleep difficulties, and mood changes, women may become less physically active during menopause. This might result in a loss of general strength and fitness.

3. Bone loss: Menopause is connected with a decrease in bone density, which can increase the risk of fractures and have an influence on overall strength. Body composition changes: There is a shift in body composition during menopause, with a loss in muscle mass and an increase in body fat. This can result in a change in general body form, with more fat accumulating around the waist and abdomen.

4. Vaginal alterations: Menopause can also induce vaginal tissue changes, such as thinning and reduced suppleness. This might lead to a sense of diminished pelvic support, which can influence overall body form. There is less desire for sex. Dryness (loss of libido) and soreness, itching, or discomfort during intercourse are examples of vaginal alterations.

5. Breast alterations: Menopause can lead to changes in breast tissue, including a loss of firmness and flexibility.
6. Changes in metabolism: Menopause can also be related to changes in metabolism, such as a decline in basal metabolic rate, which can result in weight gain.

A good diet and regular physical activity can help reduce some of the effects of menopause on body shape. Resistance training and weight-bearing exercises can aid in the maintenance of muscle mass and bone density, whereas cardiovascular exercise can aid in the maintenance of general fitness and the prevention of weight gain. Wearing supportive undergarments can also assist to preserve excellent posture and a young body shape.

CHAPTER 6

Is it just me, it is hot in here? Vasomotor Symptoms and How to Put Out the Fire?

Menopausal hot flashes and nocturnal sweats are examples of vasomotor symptoms (VMS). These unexpected bouts of heat and sweat may occur in women during and after the menopausal transition, when hormone levels change. VMS in menopause is caused by decreased and fluctuating hormone levels. While the specific mechanism is unknown, experts suspect that lower estrogen levels may lead your body's temperature control (the hypothalamus in the brain) to become more sensitive. Certain women are more prone to heat flashes than others. Among the risk factors are:

1. Smoking. Smoking can also lead to the development of vasomotor symptoms in menopausal women. Smoking can impair the function of blood vessels and the neurological system, resulting in alterations in body temperature regulation. Nicotine, a substance present in tobacco, can cause blood vessels to tighten, limiting blood flow to the skin and other organs. This might cause a sensation of being chilled. When blood vessels contract and then dilate, a quick and unexpected increase in blood flow can occur, resulting in a sense of being hot or a hot flash. Smoking can also impair the functioning of the hypothalamus, the portion of the brain responsible for regulating body temperature. Nicotine can cause the production of certain hormones, such as adrenaline and noradrenaline, which can alter the hypothalamus and cause changes in body temperature regulation. This can lead to the development of hot flashes and other vasomotor symptoms. Furthermore, smoking might contribute to other variables that can cause vasomotor symptoms during menopause. For instance, smoking has been linked to higher-than-average levels of anxiety and stress, which can exacerbate hot flashes and other symptoms. Smoking can also impair sleep quality, which can lead to the development of night sweats. Smoking, through its impact on blood vessel function, the neurological system, and other physiological processes, might lead to the development of vasomotor symptoms in menopausal women. Quitting smoking can help reduce the intensity and frequency of these symptoms as well as improve general health throughout menopause.

2. The emergence of vasomotor symptoms is also influenced by obesity. Obesity is defined as an excess of body fat, and it is related to a range of physiological abnormalities that might impact hormone control and body temperature. Obesity can contribute to the development of vasomotor symptoms by altering sex hormone levels. Adipose tissue, or fat tissue, generates estrogen, which can result in an overabundance of estrogen in the body in obese women. Obese women, while having greater amounts of estrogen, might develop vasomotor symptoms owing to an imbalance between estrogen and other hormones. This imbalance can interfere with body temperature control and lead to the development of hot flashes and other vasomotor symptoms. It can also cause insulin resistance, a disease in which the body is less receptive to insulin, a hormone that regulates blood sugar levels. Insulin resistance can cause increased inflammation and oxidative stress, which can impair the function of the hypothalamus, a portion of the brain that regulates body temperature. This can lead to the development of hot flashes and other vasomotor symptoms. Obesity is frequently connected with other variables that might contribute to the development of vasomotor symptoms during menopause. Obese women, for example, may be more prone to sleep apnea, a disease in which breathing is disrupted during sleep, which can contribute to the development of night sweats. Obesity is also linked to higher levels of stress and anxiety, which can worsen hot flashes and other symptoms. Obesity can contribute to the development of vasomotor symptoms in menopausal women by influencing sex hormone levels, insulin resistance, and other physiological processes. Maintaining a healthy weight and engaging in regular physical exercise can help reduce the intensity and frequency of these symptoms and improve overall health throughout menopause.

3. Stress can also lead to the development of vasomotor symptoms in menopausal women.

Stress can impair the functioning of the hypothalamus, a region of the brain responsible for regulating body temperature, by increasing the activity of the sympathetic nervous system. The sympathetic nervous system is in charge of the "fight or flight" reaction and can raise heart rate, blood pressure, and body temperature. When the sympathetic nervous system is stimulated, it can cause hot flashes and other vasomotor symptoms. Stress can also impair the function of the adrenal glands, which generate hormones such as adrenaline and cortisol. Adrenaline can raise heart rate and blood pressure, but cortisol can influence blood sugar management and immunological function.

The release of these hormones in response to stress can impair hypothalamic function and contribute to the development of vasomotor symptoms. It can also have an impact on sleep quality, which can lead to the development of night sweats. Sleep disruptions can interfere with the body's temperature regulation, resulting in perspiration and overheating. Stress can contribute to the development of vasomotor symptoms in menopausal women by influencing the sympathetic nervous system, adrenal gland function, and sleep quality. Reducing stress via relaxation techniques such as deep breathing,

meditation, or yoga can help to reduce the intensity and frequency of these symptoms while also improving general health throughout menopause.

3. Anxiety is another influence.

Anxiety can contribute to the development of vasomotor symptoms in menopausal women by influencing the sympathetic nervous system, hormone levels, and sleep quality. It has the potential to impair the functioning of the hypothalamus, a region of the brain responsible for controlling body temperature. Anxiety affects the sympathetic nervous system, which causes a rise in heart rate, blood pressure, and body temperature. When the sympathetic nervous system is stimulated, it can cause hot flashes and other vasomotor symptoms. Anxiety can change hormone levels, which can lead to the development of vasomotor symptoms. Stress chemicals such as cortisol can disrupt the body's sex hormone balance. In menopausal women, estrogen levels are already decreasing, and anxiety might aggravate this loss. Estrogen regulates body temperature, and a drop in estrogen levels can cause hot flashes and nocturnal sweats. Anxiety can also cause sleep problems, which can contribute to the development of vasomotor symptoms. Anxiety and stress can make it difficult to fall or remain asleep, resulting in poor sleep quality. Sleep disruptions can interfere with the body's temperature regulation, resulting in perspiration and overheating. Managing anxiety via relaxation methods, counseling, and lifestyle modifications can help to reduce the intensity and frequency of these symptoms while also improving overall health throughout menopause.

Why do Black Women have a Higher Risk of Vasomotor Symptoms than White Women?

According to research, black women had a greater risk of vasomotor symptoms such as hot flashes and night sweats during menopause than white women. Several variables contribute to this discrepancy, including genetics, lifestyle choices, and socioeconomic background.

To begin, genetics may play a role in the increased occurrence of vasomotor symptoms in black women. Black women have lower amounts of estradiol, a kind of estrogen, than White women, which may lead to a higher risk of vasomotor symptoms. Genetic differences in estrogen-metabolizing enzymes may potentially have a role.

Smoking, food, and physical activity may contribute to the greater prevalence of vasomotor symptoms in black women. According to research, black women are more likely to smoke and have a greater incidence of obesity, both of which are risk factors for vasomotor symptoms. A diet heavy in fat and poor in fruits and vegetables has also been linked to an increased incidence of these symptoms.

Again, socioeconomic status may play a role in the increased occurrence of vasomotor symptoms among black women. Black women are more likely to be poor and to suffer higher amounts of stress, both of which might contribute to the development of these symptoms. Furthermore, black women may find it more challenging to effectively manage their symptoms due to a lack of healthcare access and insufficient resources.

Finally, the increased frequency of vasomotor symptoms in black women following menopause is most likely attributable to a combination of genetic, lifestyle, and socioeconomic variables. More study is needed to completely understand these discrepancies and create appropriate treatments to promote the health and well-being of black women throughout menopause. Abuse History According to a preliminary study, early-life maltreatment or financial difficulty are associated with greater menopausal symptoms.

Is it possible to cure Vasomotor Symptoms?

Yes, vasomotor symptoms, which are typical in menopausal women, may be treated. There are various methods for addressing these symptoms, including lifestyle modifications, drugs, and alternative therapy.

Lifestyle adjustments can help reduce the intensity and frequency of vasomotor symptoms. These include avoiding stressors like hot meals and alcohol, keeping a healthy weight, and engaging in regular exercise. Relaxation practices such as yoga, meditation, and deep breathing exercises can also help reduce stress and manage these symptoms.

A healthcare professional may also prescribe medications to treat vasomotor symptoms. Hormone therapy, which involves taking estrogen or a combination of estrogen and progesterone, is the most effective treatment for these symptoms.

However, hormone treatment is not suited for many women and may have certain hazards, so it should be reviewed with a healthcare practitioner to decide if it is the best option.

Other drugs, such as selective serotonin reuptake inhibitors (SSRIs) and gabapentin, may also be used to treat similar symptoms .Acupuncture and herbal supplements, for example, may be beneficial in controlling vasomotor symptoms. More study, however, is required to completely understand the effectiveness and safety of these medicines.

It is crucial to remember that vasomotor symptoms can vary in severity and duration among individuals, and what works for one woman may not work for another. It is suggested that women experiencing these symptoms consult with their healthcare professionals about the best alternatives for managing their symptoms based on their unique requirements and medical history.

VSM therapy options include:

1. Hormone Therapy

Hormone therapy (HT) is the most effective treatment for vasomotor symptoms. The risks differ from woman to woman, so make sure you have a detailed conversation with your healthcare provider about your specific requirements. You might also consult a menopausal specialist, who has additional training in how to care for you during your menopause transition.

2. Nonhormonal Therapy

If you cannot or do not want to take HT, there are other non-hormonal alternatives. Some researchers have seen effectiveness with oxybutynin (Ditropan), GABAergic, clonidine (Catapres), selective serotonin reuptake inhibitors, and selective serotonin-norepinephrine reuptake inhibitors. More are being developed. Again, consult with your doctor about the best option for you.

3. Lifestyle changes

According to research, the benefits of some lifestyle modifications only exacerbate menopausal symptoms. It is recommended that you stop smoking and drinking alcohol, drink cold beverages, and pour cool water over your face and wrists. Also, keep an eye on your weight. Hot flushes have been linked to body mass index in studies. You can also wear it in layers to avoid temperature changes.

4. Diet and Dietary Changes

Caffeine, spicy meals, hot beverages, and processed sugar (candy, cookies, and cakes) are all known to cause or worsen hot flashes. Soy foods and natural soy products such as tofu. Avoid highly processed soy foods that are heavy in salt, sugar, unhealthy fats, additives, and fillers. Foods high in omega-3 fatty acids. Salmon, mackerel, tuna, herring, sardines, and other cold-water fatty fish are all included. Plant-based meals are an essential component of Mediterranean diet. The Mediterranean Diet has been demonstrated to minimize the incidence of hot flashes due to its concentration of vegetables, fruits, nuts, legumes, seeds, olive oil, and fish, as well as its moderate usage of dairy and reduced consumption of red meat. Instead, try to load your plate with these potential hot flash reducers.

5. Breathing exercises may assist with VMS symptoms

Breathing exercises can assist control the body's reaction and minimize the severity of symptoms. One breathing activity that may be useful is deep breathing or diaphragmatic breathing. This entails breathing deeply and slowly from the diaphragm, rather than shallowly from the chest. To practice this, sit comfortably with your back straight and your hands resting on your stomach. Inhale deeply through your nose, filling your lungs with air and extending your belly. Exhale gently via your lips, emptying your lungs and compressing your belly. Repeat this pattern for many minutes, concentrating on your breath and relaxing your body. Another breathing practice that may be useful is timed breathing, which includes breathing at a slow and constant rate. To practice this, inhale deeply for a count of four, hold your breath for a count of four, and then exhale gently for a count of four. Repeat this pattern for many minutes, concentrating on your breath and relaxing your body. Breathing exercises can help reduce stress and worry, which can increase vasomotor symptoms and also help regulate the body's temperature.

6. VSM symptoms can be managed with stress-reduction techniques.

Stress reduction can be effective in controlling vasomotor symptoms (VMS) because stress can increase these symptoms. Stress causes the body's "fight or flight" reaction, which can produce a rise in heart rate, blood pressure, and body temperature. These physiological alterations might contribute to hot flashes and nocturnal sweats. Stress reduction approaches, such as relaxation techniques, mindfulness, and physical activity, can assist to lessen the body's stress response and increase general well-being. Relaxation techniques, such as deep breathing, gradual muscle relaxation, and visualization, can assist to calm the body and relieve stress.

CHAPTER 7
Menstrual Mayhem: Abnormal Bleedings and How to Deal with It.

The most prevalent causes of bleeding or spotting after menopause include:
1. Endometrial or vaginal atrophy (the lining of the uterus or vagina becomes thin and dry).
Hormone replacement treatment (HRT) (estrogen and progesterone pills that alleviate some menopausal symptoms).
Uterine cancer or endometrial cancer (cancer in the lining of the uterus).
Endometrial hyperplasia (the lining of the uterus grows overly thick and might include aberrant cells).
Uterine polyps (growths in the uterus).
Other factors might include:
Cervical cancer (carcinoma in the cervix). Cervicitis or endometritis (infection or inflammation in the cervix or uterus).
Bleeding from other regions, nearby, in the bladder or rectum or bleeding from the skin of the vulva (outside near the vagina)
Medication and surgery are the most popular treatments. They include:
1. Antibiotics can treat most infections of the cervix or uterus.
2. Estrogen may improve bleeding due to vaginal dryness. You can administer estrogen straight to your vagina as a cream, ring or insertable pill. Systemic estrogen treatment may come as a tablet or patch. When estrogen treatment is systemic, it implies the hormone goes throughout the body.
3. Progestin is a synthetic version of the hormone progesterone. It can cure endometrial hyperplasia by prompting the uterus to shed its lining. You may get progestin as a tablet, injection, cream or intrauterine device (IUD).
Surgeries include:
1. *Hysteroscopy* is a treatment to check your cervix and uterus with a camera. Your healthcare professional inserts a hysteroscope (thin, lighted tube) into your vagina to remove polyps or other abnormal growths that may be causing bleeding. This can be done in the office for diagnosis. To remove any growths, hysteroscopy is generally done in the operating room under general anesthesia.
2. Dilation and curettage (D&C) is a technique to sample the lining and contents of the uterus. Your healthcare professional may conduct a D&C with a hysteroscopy. A D&C can treat some kinds of endometrial hyperplasia.
Will I still suffer Menopause if I have gone through Hysterectomy?

Hysterectomy is a procedure to remove your uterus and cervix. You may need a hysterectomy if you have uterine cancer. If you have undergone a hysterectomy, which is the surgical removal of the uterus, you will no longer experience menstrual cycles since you no longer have a uterus. However, whether or not you will still experience menopause depends on whether or not your ovaries were also removed during the procedure.

If your ovaries were not removed during the hysterectomy, you may still experience menopause when your ovaries naturally cease releasing eggs and hormones, which normally occurs in the late 40s or early 50s for most women. The symptoms of menopause might include hot flashes, mood changes, vaginal dryness, and other changes connected with the drop in estrogen levels.

If your ovaries were removed during the hysterectomy, you will have surgical menopause, which can arrive rapidly and may have more severe symptoms than natural menopause. In this instance, your body will quickly cease manufacturing hormones, and you may suffer symptoms including hot flashes, night sweats, vaginal dryness, and mood problems.

It is crucial to explore the potential repercussions of a hysterectomy with your doctor before the operation to completely understand what to expect and how it may affect your health and well-being.

CHAPTER 8

Now concerning the Vagina and Vulva: Genitourinary Syndrome of Menopause and the Therapies. Let's speak about Sex.; The Complex Story of Desire during Menopause.

Genitourinary syndrome of menopause (GSM) is characterized as a combination of symptoms and indicators induced by hypoestrogenic alterations to the labia majora/minora, clitoris, vestibule/introitus, vagina, urethra, and bladder that occur in menopausal individuals. Genitourinary Syndrome of Menopause (GSM) is a disorder that affects many women throughout menopause. GSM refers to a set of symptoms that are induced by the falling levels of estrogen in a woman's body during menopause. As estrogen levels decline, the tissues of the vagina, vulva, and urinary system become thinner, less elastic, and more brittle, which can contribute to a range of unpleasant and even painful symptoms. Some frequent symptoms of GSM include vaginal dryness, itching, burning, discomfort during intercourse, and urine incontinence. These symptoms can have a substantial influence on a woman's quality of life, including discomfort, agony, and humiliation.

Helpful Treatments:

Fortunately, there are various treatment options available for GSM that can help ease symptoms and enhance the quality of life. One of the most prevalent treatments for GSM is hormone therapy, which entails utilizing estrogen to augment the body's natural levels and promote vaginal and urinary tract health. Hormone treatment can be taken orally, through a patch, or as a vaginal cream or ring. To treat the genitourinary syndrome of menopause, your doctor may first offer over-the-counter medication alternatives, including:

1. Vaginal moisturizers

Try a vaginal moisturizer (K-Y Liquibase, Replens, etc.) to restore some moisture to your vaginal region. You may have to use the moisturizer every few days. The benefits of a moisturizer often linger a bit longer than those of a lubricant.

Water-based lubricants. These lubricants (Astro Glide, K-Y Jelly, etc.) are used soon before sexual activity and help lessen pain during intercourse. Choose products that don't include glycerin or warming characteristics since women who are sensitive to these compounds may feel discomfort. Avoid petroleum jelly or other petroleum-based items for lubrication if you're also using condoms because petroleum can break down latex condoms on contact.

2. Topical estrogen

Vaginal estrogen has the benefit of being effective at lower levels and reducing your overall exposure to estrogen because less reaches your bloodstream. It may also provide greater direct alleviation of symptoms than oral estrogen does. Vaginal estrogen treatment comes in a number of forms. Because they all seem to function equally well, you and your doctor can determine which one is best for you. Vaginal estrogen cream (Estrace, Premarin). You apply this cream straight into your vagina using an applicator, generally at night. Typically, women use it daily for one to three weeks and then one to three times a week thereafter, but your doctor will let you know how much cream to use and how often to insert it.

Vaginal estrogen suppositories (Imvexy). These low-dose estrogen suppositories are injected around 2 inches into the vaginal canal, for weeks. Then, the suppositories only need to be inserted twice a week. Vaginal estrogen ring (Estring, Femring). A soft, flexible ring is inserted into the upper region of the vagina by you or your doctor. The ring provides a steady amount of estrogen while in place and has to be changed around every three months. Many ladies prefer the convenience this affords. A new, higher dosage ring is considered a systemic rather than topical therapy.

Vaginal estrogen pill (Vagifem). You use a disposable applicator to implant a vaginal estrogen pill in your vagina. Your doctor will let you know how often to inject the medication. You may, for instance, use it daily for the first two weeks and then twice a week thereafter.

3. Ospemifene (Osphena).

Taken daily, this medication can help reduce unpleasant sexual symptoms in women with moderate to severe GSM. It is not authorized in women who've had breast cancer or who have a high risk of getting breast cancer.

4. Prasterone (Intrarosa).

These vaginal inserts release the hormone DHEA straight to the vagina to assist relieve painful intercourse. DHEA is a hormone that helps the body generate other hormones, including estrogen. Prasterone is taken nightly for moderate-to-severe vaginal atrophy.

5. Systemic estrogen treatment

If vaginal dryness is linked with additional symptoms of menopause, such as moderate or severe hot flashes, your doctor may advise estrogen tablets, patches or gel, or a higher dosage estrogen ring. Estrogen taken by mouth reaches your complete system. Ask your doctor to clarify the dangers vs. advantages of oral estrogen, and whether or not you would also need to take another hormone called progestin along with estrogen.

6. Vaginal dilators

You may utilize vaginal dilators as a nonhormonal therapy alternative. Vaginal dilators may also be utilized in conjunction with estrogen treatment. These devices stimulate and expand the vaginal muscles to reverse the constriction of the vagina. If painful sex is an issue, vaginal dilators may ease vaginal discomfort by extending the vagina. They are accessible without a prescription, but if your symptoms are severe, your doctor may recommend pelvic floor physical therapy and vaginal dilators. Your healthcare practitioner or a pelvic physical therapist can show you how to utilize vaginal dilators.

7. Topical lidocaine

Available as a prescription ointment or gel, topical lidocaine can be used to decrease the discomfort associated with sexual activity. Apply it five to 10 minutes before you begin sexual activity.

For more severe cases of GSM, laser therapy or surgery may be recommended.

Laser treatment can be used to treat GSM by stimulating collagen formation and repairing vaginal tissue. This therapy includes the use of a customized laser that provides regulated energy to the vaginal tissue, encouraging the formation of collagen and elastin. Laser therapy may be administered in an outpatient environment, and it normally takes less than 30 minutes to complete. During the process, a tiny probe is introduced into the vagina, and laser energy is given to the vaginal tissue. The therapy is painless and requires no anesthetic or downtime. Laser therapy can assist to rebuild vaginal tissue, enhancing suppleness, lubrication, and blood flow to the region. This can assist to reduce symptoms such as vaginal dryness, itching, and burning, as well as uncomfortable intercourse. Laser therapy can be an effective and non-invasive therapeutic option for women with GSM.

Surgery.

Surgery is not a popular therapeutic option for genitourinary syndrome of menopause (GSM). However, several surgical treatments may be advised in specific instances. One surgical treatment for treating GSM is vaginal rejuvenation surgery. This process includes the use of a laser or radiofrequency device to promote collagen formation in the vaginal tissue, which can help restore vaginal health and reduce symptoms such as vaginal dryness, itching, and painful intercourse.

Another surgical option is a vaginal hysterectomy. In rare situations, a hysterectomy may be suggested to manage diseases such as uterine prolapse or cervical cancer. During this surgery, the uterus is removed, which can ease the strain on the vaginal walls and enhance vaginal health.

Let's speak about Sex. The Complex Story of Desire during Menopause.
Fluctuating menopausal hormone levels and menopause symptoms might wreak havoc with your enthusiasm for sex. Some women endure vaginal dryness when their bodies encounter the change. This can make sex painful. Women may also suffer a tightness of the vaginal opening, burning, itching, and dryness (called vaginal atrophy). Fortunately, there are choices for women to address these difficulties. However, not all women go through this libido decline, but it is fairly prevalent. Various variables might lead to a decline in sexual desire or libido in women during menopause:

1. Hormonal changes: Menopause is connected with a decline in the production of estrogen and testosterone, which can influence sexual desire and arousal.

2. Physical changes: Menopause can also induce physical changes that might influence sexual activity, including vaginal dryness, weakening of vaginal tissues, and a loss in natural lubrication.

3. Psychological factors: Menopause may be a tough period for many women, and it can be accompanied by feelings of worry, melancholy, and stress. These variables can alter sexual desire and function.

4. Relationship difficulties: Changes in sexual desire and function can occasionally lead to relationship troubles, which can further influence libido. It is crucial to highlight that a reduction in sexual desire after menopause is typical, and it does not necessarily imply a disease or anomaly. However, if the drop in libido is causing discomfort or compromising the quality of life, it may be worth discussing with a healthcare physician. Treatment methods may include hormonal therapy, counselling is also suggested for couples with relationship issues whether or not it directly impacts their sexual life or other techniques to promote sexual health and well-being.

CHAPTER 9
Cardiovascular Symptoms and Therapies.

Do menopausal women have an increased risk of cardiovascular disease?
A substantial amount of research has related menopause with cardiovascular disease, including risk factors such as increased LDL (bad cholesterol) and decreasing HDL (good cholesterol). Plus, studies that have followed women over a length of time have indicated that those women with early menopause (45 and younger) had greater cardiovascular health difficulties later on than those who experience menopause closer to the typical age (about 50).

Complex hormonal changes are taking place during menopause, particularly when menopause occurs at a younger age compared to the normal menopausal age of 50 years. Early menopause seems to have some influence on cardiovascular health, but there is still lots of controversy as to exactly what that effect is and how much.

Also, many cardiovascular issues that are related to menopause might be attributable to ordinary aging.

Hormone Therapy (HRT)
During menopause, the ovaries progressively stop generating estrogen. Hormone replacement treatment (HRT) is a means to give part of the estrogen back and assist manage typical menopausal symptoms such as hot flashes, as well as prevent osteoporosis. Estrogen drugs are frequently taken orally as a tablet, applied to the skin via a cream or a patch, or administered intravaginally.

Taken alone, estrogen can raise a woman's likelihood of getting endometrial cancer (cancer in the uterine lining). During a woman's pre-menopausal and reproductive years, menstruation causes the body to lose endometrial cells. During menopause, this stops occurring, and injecting estrogen might trigger an excess of these cells.

Estrogen is commonly administered alongside progesterone to decrease or reverse the proliferation of endometrial cells. For women who have undergone hysterectomies, this proliferation of cells is not a concern, therefore estrogen is administered by itself.

What effect does hormone replacement treatment have on cardiovascular health?

Hormone replacement treatment can be effective in treating menopausal symptoms (hot flashes, etc.) and helping to avoid osteoporosis. But there's still dispute as to its cardiovascular advantages. There are numerous new research now studying the difference between women who receive hormone replacement closer to menopause vs. later in life.

Based on the present data, the FDA recommends that women who take hormone replacement therapy do so under strict physician supervision, and exclusively for controlling menopausal symptoms such as hot flashes. Women are not encouraged to utilize hormone replacement treatment for decreasing cardiovascular risk.

Menopause involves the whole body and may call for more than a gynecologist's care. The hormonal changes that occur during menopause can bring greater cardiovascular risk in the form of elevated blood pressure and cholesterol levels.

If cardiovascular disease runs strongly in the family, you must consult a cardiologist to further analyze the chance of getting cardiovascular disease and to maximize therapy

CHAPTER 10
Osteoporosis with Menopause, Treatment and Prevention.

Osteoporosis is a condition that weakens bones, increasing the risk of abrupt and unexpected fractures. Meaning "porous bone," osteoporosis leads to an increasing loss of bone mass and strength. The illness generally advances without any signs or discomfort.

Many often, osteoporosis is not identified until weakening bones cause painful fractures commonly in the back or hips. Unfortunately, if you have a fractured bone due to osteoporosis, you are at great risk of having another. And these fractures can be devastating. Fortunately, there are things you may do to help prevent osteoporosis from ever happening. And therapies can delay the pace of bone loss if you already have osteoporosis.

What Causes Osteoporosis?
Though scientists may not know the specific origin of osteoporosis, we do know how the illness progresses. Your bones are formed of life, developing tissue. An outer shell of cortical or thick bone encases trabecular bone, a sponge-like bone. When a bone is affected by osteoporosis, the "holes" in the "sponge" get larger and more frequent, damaging the internal structure of the bone.

Until roughly age 30, humans generally create more bone than they lose. During the aging process, bone breakdown begins to outstrip bone growth, resulting in a steady decrease in bone mass. Once this loss of bone reaches a particular threshold, a person has osteoporosis.

How Is Osteoporosis Related to Menopause?
There is a clear association between the loss of estrogen during perimenopause and menopause and the development of osteoporosis. Early menopause (before age 45) and any protracted periods in which hormone levels are low and menstrual cycles are absent or uncommon might cause loss of bone density.

What Are the Symptoms of Osteoporosis?
Osteoporosis is frequently dubbed a "silent disease" since initially bone loss happens without symptoms. People may not realize that they have osteoporosis until their bones become so weak that a sudden strain, jolt, or tumble causes a fracture or a vertebra to collapse. Collapsed vertebrae may initially be felt or seen in the form of acute back discomfort, loss of height, or spinal abnormalities such as stooped posture.

How Do I Know I Have Osteoporosis?

A painless and reliable test can reveal information about bone health and osteoporosis before issues develop. Bone mineral density (BMD) examinations, or bone measures, are X-rays that employ extremely tiny levels of radiation to detect bone strength.

A bone mineral density test is advised for: women age 65 and older, women with several risk factors, and menopausal women who have had fractures

How Is Osteoporosis Treated?

Treatments for established osteoporosis (meaning, you already have osteoporosis) include: • Medications such as alendronate (Binosto, Fosamax), ibandronate (Boniva), raloxifene (Evista), risedronate (Actonel, Atevia), and zoledronic acid (Reclast, Zometa)

• Calcium and vitamin D supplements.

• Weight-bearing workouts (which make your muscles work against gravity)

• Injectable abaloparatide (Tymlos), teriparatide (Forteo) or PTH to restore bone

• Injectable denosumab (Prolia, Xgeva) for women at high risk of fracture when other medications don't work • Hormone therapy

Should I Consider Hormone Therapy?

Hormone treatment [estrogen] is considered to be beneficial in preventing or reducing the accelerated rate of bone loss that leads to osteoporosis. However, utilizing hormone replacement therapy for the prevention of osteoporosis alone—not to relieve menopausal symptoms—is not advised by the FDA.

If you are using hormone treatment exclusively for osteoporosis prevention, be careful to talk to your doctor so you can assess the advantages of hormone therapy against your particular risk and explore other drugs for your bones. If required, your doctor might prescribe several therapies to help prevent osteoporosis.

Is There a Safe Alternative to Hormone Therapy?

Alternatives to hormone treatment include • Bisphosphonates. This category of pharmaceuticals comprises the drugs alendronate (Binosto, Fosamax), risedronate (Actonel, Atelvia), ibandronate (Boniva) and zoledronic acid (Reclast, Zometa). Bisphosphonates are used to prevent and/or cure osteoporosis. All can help avoid spine fractures. Binosto, Fosamax, Actonel, Atelvia, Reclast and Zometa can help lower the risk of hip and other non-spine fractures.

• Raloxifene (Evista). This medicine is a selective estrogen receptor modulator (SERM) that has numerous estrogen-like characteristics. It is licensed for prevention and treatment of osteoporosis and can prevent bone loss in the spine, hip, and other

parts of the body. Studies have indicated that it can lower the rate of vertebral fractures by 30%-50%. It may raise the risk of blood clots.
• Teriparatide (Forteo) and Tymlos, are a kind of hormone used to treat osteoporosis. They help regenerate bone and boost bone mineral density. They are delivered by injection and are used as a therapy for osteoporosis.
• Denosumab (Prolia, Xgeva) is a so-called monoclonal antibody -- a human, lab-produced antibody that inactivates the body's bone-breakdown process. It is used to treat women at high risk of fracture when other osteoporosis medications have not worked.

How Can I Prevent Osteoporosis?
There are various methods you may help protect yourself against osteoporosis, including exercise. Establish a regular workout routine. Exercise makes bones and muscles stronger and helps prevent bone loss. It also helps you keep active and mobile. Weight-bearing workouts, done at least three to four times a week, are optimal for preventing osteoporosis. Walking, running, playing tennis, and dancing are all terrific weight-bearing workouts. In addition, strength and balance workouts may help you prevent falls, lessening your probability of fracturing a bone. • Eat foods high in calcium. Getting adequate calcium throughout your life helps to create and retain healthy bones. The U.S. recommended daily amount (RDA) of calcium for people with a low-to-average risk of developing osteoporosis is 1,000 mg (milligrams) each day. For people at high risk of developing osteoporosis, such as postmenopausal women and men, the RDA climbs up to 1,200 mg each day. Excellent sources of calcium are milk and dairy products (low-fat versions are advised), tinned fish with bones like salmon and sardines, dark green leafy vegetables, such as kale, collards and broccoli, calcium-fortified orange juice, and bread prepared with calcium-fortified flour.
• Supplements. If you think you need to take a supplement to get adequate calcium, check with your doctor first. Calcium carbonate and calcium citrate are effective kinds of calcium supplementation. Be cautious not to get more than 2,000 mg of calcium a day if you are 51 or older. Younger persons may be able to handle up to 2500 mg a day but check with your doctor. Too much might raise the possibility of developing kidney stones.
• Vitamin D. Your body utilizes vitamin D to absorb calcium. Being out in the sun for a total of 20 minutes per day helps most people's bodies manufacture adequate

vitamin D. You may also acquire vitamin D via eggs, fatty seafood like salmon, cereal and milk enriched with vitamin D, as well as from supplements.

People aged 51 to 70 should receive 600 IU daily. More than 4,000 IU of vitamin D per day is not advised. Talk to your doctor to discover how much is suitable for you because it may hurt your kidneys and potentially diminish bone mass.
• Medications. Most of the bisphosphonates that are taken by mouth as well as raloxifene (Evista) can be administered to assist prevent osteoporosis in those who are at high risk for fractures.
• Estrogen. Estrogen, a hormone generated by the ovaries, helps protect against bone loss. It can be used as therapy for the prevention of osteoporosis. Replacing estrogen lost during menopause (when the ovaries halt most of their synthesis of estrogen) decreases bone loss and enhances the body's absorption and retention of calcium. But, because estrogen treatment entails hazards, it is only indicated for women at high risk for osteoporosis and/or severe menopausal symptoms. To learn more, talk to your doctor about the advantages and cons of estrogen treatment.
• Know the high-risk drugs. Steroids, some breast cancer medicines (such as aromatase inhibitors), pharmaceuticals used to treat seizures (anticonvulsants), blood thinners (anticoagulants), and thyroid medications can accelerate the rate of bone loss. If you are taking any of these medicines, chat with your doctor about ways to lower your risk of bone loss through diet, lifestyle changes and, maybe, extra medication.
• Other preventative actions. Limit alcohol consumption and do not smoke. Smoking causes your body to create less estrogen, which protects the bones. Too much alcohol can weaken your bones and raise the chance of falling and fracturing a bone.

How Can I Get the Calcium My Body Needs If I'm Lactose Intolerant
If you are lactose intolerant or have problems digesting milk, you may not be receiving enough calcium in your diet. Although most dairy products may be uncomfortable, certain yogurt and hard cheeses could be edible. You can also eat lactose-containing food by first treating it with commercial preparations of lactase (which can be added as drops or taken as tablets). There are other lactose-free dairy products you may buy. You can also eat lactose-free foods high in calcium, such as leafy green vegetables, salmon (with bones), and broccoli. There are several foods that are fortified with calcium too, such as certain orange juices and breads

Weight-Bearing Exercises and How Do They Help Strengthen Bone.

Weight-bearing workouts are activities that make your muscles work against gravity. Walking, hiking, stair-climbing, or running are all weight-bearing workouts that assist create strong bones.

Thirty minutes of regular exercise (at least 3 to 4 days a week or every other day) paired with a nutritious diet may enhance peak bone mass in younger adults. Older women and men who engage in regular exercise may see decreased bone loss or even increased bone mass.

If you have osteoporosis, it is crucial to safeguard yourself against unintentional falls, which may result in fractures. Take the following steps to make your house safe: remove loose household objects, keep your home free of clutter, install grab bars on tub and shower walls and near toilets, install appropriate lighting, apply treads to floors and remove throw rugs.

CHAPTER 11

Brain Health: Brain Fog, Depression and Dementia, Sleep Disturbances.

Brain fog is a typical symptom described by many women throughout menopause. It is characterized by feelings of bewilderment, forgetfulness, and trouble concentrating. The specific origin of brain fog during menopause is not entirely understood, however, it is considered to be connected to hormone changes and other variables. During menopause, the levels of estrogen and other hormones in the body decline. Estrogen plays a role in cognitive function, including memory and attention. When levels of estrogen decline, it can lead to changes in the brain that impact cognitive function and contribute to brain fog.

In addition to hormonal changes, several factors may contribute to brain fog during menopause. These include sleep difficulties, stress, anxiety, sadness, and drug side effects. Sleep difficulties, such as insomnia or waking up frequently throughout the night, can contribute to weariness and trouble concentrating during the day. Stress, anxiety, and sadness can also disrupt cognitive performance and contribute to brain fog. Medication side effects might also lead to cognitive fog during menopause. Certain drugs, such as antidepressants and blood pressure medications, can induce cognitive adverse effects such as disorientation and difficulties concentrating.

It is crucial to highlight that brain fog can have a substantial influence on everyday living and quality of life for women suffering from it throughout menopause.

Dementia is a word used to indicate a deterioration in cognitive function that is severe enough to interfere with daily activities. It is not considered a natural component of aging, but rather a combination of symptoms that can be caused by many underlying disorders or diseases, such as Alzheimer's disease, Parkinson's disease, or stroke. Dementia is not commonly considered a menopausal symptom, although the hormonal changes associated with menopause may contribute to cognitive impairment or raise the chance of developing dementia in some women. Specifically, research has revealed that lowering estrogen levels following menopause may be a contributing cause of cognitive impairment and an increased chance of acquiring dementia in some women. Estrogen has a protective function in brain health, and studies have indicated that women who have early menopause or have reduced estrogen levels may be at an increased risk of having cognitive impairment or dementia later in life.

Some studies have also shown that hormone treatment may be protective against cognitive impairment in some women. It is crucial to highlight, however, that the association between menopause and dementia is complicated and not entirely understood. While lowering estrogen levels may be a contributing factor, there are numerous variables that might potentially raise the risk of cognitive decline and dementia, such as genetics, lifestyle factors, and other medical problems. Depression is a typical symptom encountered by many women throughout menopause. The specific cause of depression during menopause is not entirely understood, however, it is considered to be connected to hormonal changes that occur during this period. Specifically, the reduction in estrogen levels that happens with menopause might impair mood control in certain women.

Estrogen has been found to have a favorable influence on serotonin levels in the brain, which is a neurotransmitter important for regulating mood. When estrogen levels decline, serotonin levels can also fall, which can contribute to the development of depression. Menopause is sometimes accompanied by other unpleasant experiences such as physical symptoms, changes in body image, and social role shifts, which can significantly impair a woman's mental health. Women may suffer stress, worry, and loss during this period, which might raise the chance of developing depression. In addition to hormonal changes and external pressures, a personal or family history of depression as well as other mental health conditions may increase the risk of developing depression after menopause.

How to Handle Them

Midlife is a turning point, and there are many things you can do to support brain function which may include:

1. Eating a healthy diet.

There are established linkages between what we consume and our hormone balance. A brain-friendly diet is one high in polyunsaturated fatty acids, such as Omega 3 and Omega 6, which are found in eggs, fish, nuts, and seeds. Other items that may be good include fruits, vegetables, whole grains, and lean meats. A healthy diet can help keep blood sugar levels stable and supply the necessary nutrients, both of which reduce brain fog symptoms. Consuming meals with a high glycemic index, such as sugary foods and processed carbs, can cause blood sugar levels to jump and then plummet, leading to feelings of exhaustion and difficulty concentrating. Consuming a well-balanced diet rich in protein, fiber, and complex carbohydrates will aid in stabilizing blood sugar levels and preventing these oscillations. Maintaining a healthy weight through a balanced diet helps minimize the chance of developing various health disorders that might contribute to brain fog, such as high blood pressure, diabetes, and heart disease. Another crucial nutritional concern is feeding your brain antioxidants, in particular vitamins A, C and E.

The brain is the most metabolically active organ in the body. When it consumes glucose, free radicals are created which have undesirable consequences in your body, including the brain, since they cause your cells to age quicker and perform less efficiently. It's crucial to include antioxidants in your diet since they may balance out these free radicals and decrease the detrimental impact on your cells. A balanced diet can help lessen symptoms of brain fog during menopause by supplying required nutrients, maintaining stable blood sugar levels, and minimizing the chance of developing other health disorders

2. Exercise regularly.
Regular exercise can also improve brain health. It is crucial to create time to remain active by performing an activity that you like. If you're not keen on going to the gym or taking a fitness class, yoga is a terrific way to reduce tension and encourage relaxation. Going for a regular stroll can enhance fitness and promote mental and emotional wellness. Regular exercise has been found to provide several physical and mental health advantages, including lowering symptoms of brain fog during menopause. Brain fog is a frequent symptom reported by many women throughout menopause, characterized by difficulties concentrating, forgetfulness, and disorientation. Although the specific origin of brain fog during menopause is not completely known, it is considered to be connected to hormonal changes that occur during this period. It can help minimize symptoms of brain fog by improving blood flow and oxygen to the brain, stimulating the creation of new brain cells, and lowering inflammation in the body. Exercise has also been demonstrated to boost mood, reduce stress and anxiety, and promote self-esteem, all of which can positively benefit cognitive performance. Hormones that can cause brain fog during menopause can be controlled with exercise. For example, exercise has been proven to enhance levels of endorphins, which are substances that can improve mood and lessen pain. Exercise can also help control cortisol levels, which are stress chemicals that can interfere with cognitive function. It can also help maintain a healthy weight and minimize the chance of developing other health disorders that can contribute to brain fog, such as high blood pressure, diabetes, and heart disease. Regular exercise can help reduce symptoms of brain fog during menopause by increasing blood flow and oxygen to the brain, promoting the growth of new brain cells, reducing inflammation, regulating hormones, improving mood, reducing stress and anxiety, increasing self-esteem, maintaining a healthy weight, and reducing the risk of developing other health conditions. It is crucial to

talk with a healthcare practitioner before starting a new fitness regimen to identify the most effective strategy for individual needs during menopause.

It can be tough to start a new eating and fitness regimen, especially if you're coping with menopausal symptoms. The objective is to create incremental, durable improvements that become part of your normal habit. Many women feel that their energy and enthusiasm to exercise increase after they start on HRT.

3. Deep sleep helps improve brain health.
It is typical to have difficulties sleeping throughout perimenopause and menopause since the brain can't regulate sleep correctly without the hormones, estrogen and progesterone. If you struggle to get or remain asleep, or you wake up in the middle of the night, there's a strong chance you're losing out on some of the deep sleep, that's most useful for your brain. Deep sleep is essential for maintaining a healthy brain because it is during this period of sleep that all toxins and impurities are flushed from the body. Because of this, it is advisable to try to improve your sleeping habits, such as reducing screen time before bed, keeping your bedroom cool, cozy, and dark, and using pillow sprays or aromatherapy oils to encourage a calm, relaxed state of mind. Many women report that the quality of their sleep substantially improves after they begin taking HRT. Additionally, getting more sleep improves mood, energy, and attention, which helps the brain fog lift. throughout deep sleep, the brain consolidates memories and processes information gained throughout the day, which can boost cognitive performance and lessen symptoms of brain fog. Additionally, deep sleep has been proven to increase immunological function, reduce inflammation, and promote tissue regeneration, all of which can positively benefit cognitive performance and lessen brain fog. However, many women have disturbances in their sleep habits after menopause, including trouble getting asleep, staying asleep, and obtaining deep sleep. This disturbance can increase feelings of brain fog and lead to daytime weariness and impaired cognitive performance. There are several strategies that women can use to improve their sleep quality during menopause, including creating a relaxing sleep environment, avoiding caffeine and alcohol before bedtime, establishing a consistent sleep routine, and practicing relaxation techniques such as deep breathing or meditation. In certain situations, women may also benefit from hormone treatment or other medical measures to increase sleep quality and lessen symptoms of brain fog. Deep sleep has a key role in cognitive function and memory consolidation, and disturbances in sleep patterns during menopause can contribute to symptoms of brain fog. Strategies to increase sleep quality, such as providing a soothing sleep environment and practicing relaxation methods, can

help lessen symptoms of brain fog and improve general cognitive performance during menopause.

4. Being positive-minded.
This decreases the load on the brain from anxiety and despair. Sound sleep aids in the correct functioning of the brain. For a decent sleep, you have to go to bed with positive thoughts, wanting to attain your ambitions and dreaming about a better tomorrow. Positive thinking may be a helpful strategy for controlling symptoms of brain fog during menopause. Brain fog is a frequent symptom reported by many women throughout menopause, characterized by difficulties concentrating, forgetfulness, and disorientation.

Although the specific origin of brain fog during menopause is not completely known, it is considered to be connected to hormonal changes that occur during this period. Negative thoughts and emotions, such as worry, anxiety, and irritation, can increase symptoms of brain fog and interfere with cognitive performance. In contrast, positive thoughts and emotions, such as optimism, hope, and thankfulness, can reduce stress and boost mood, which can positively influence cognitive performance. One technique to foster positive thinking is via mindfulness activities, such as meditation or deep breathing exercises. These activities can help relax the mind and reduce stress, allowing for better thinking and increased cognitive performance. Another strategy to encourage positive thinking is to focus on appreciation and happiness in daily life. This might entail maintaining a gratitude notebook, committing acts of kindness, or surrounding oneself with good people and experiences. By concentrating on the positive in life, women may change their attitude away from negative ideas and emotions, which can enhance cognitive performance and minimize symptoms of brain fog. It is crucial to remember that positive thinking alone may not be enough to erase symptoms of brain fog during menopause. Other techniques, like keeping a balanced diet, frequent exercise, and obtaining appropriate restful sleep, may also be important to control symptoms and enhance cognitive performance.

Positive thinking along with techniques such as good nutrition, regular exercise, and restful sleep are comprehensive tools for controlling menopausal symptoms. Midlife is a turning moment, and there are many things you can do to support brain function.

CHAPTER 12
After Menopause, What Next?

After menopause, there are numerous ways to add value to your life and enjoy this new part of your journey. Remember that menopause is just another chapter in your life narrative. Embrace the changes, keep happy, and continue to find opportunities to develop and enjoy everything that life has to offer. Here are a few suggestions:

Give back what you have.
Have you considered speaking to groups, young people or even your fellow menopausal ladies about your life experiences and lesson you have gained so far What about the fulfillment from dramatically touching people in an hour or 30-minute speech? Sometimes, we wonder what we have to contribute, but that query would be answered after expressing a few sentences. Your life narrative might be the answer to most questions individuals ask themselves. You do not only teach others, but you also learn from the comments, opinions, and even queries of your audience. It might not be a personal meeting, but virtual meetings can be regarded as such. Volunteer your time and skills to benefit others. This might be a terrific way to feel satisfied and give back to your community.

Are you pleased with your retirement account?
The dissatisfaction of not being able to save or invest enough for the future generation is frequent among menopausal women. This is a key contributing factor to the degree of sadness or anxiety in women above age 40. Therefore, it is advisable to control this by considering the following ways:

1. Find jobs that offer flexible schedules.

During your menopausal stage, it is advised to minimize stress and relax more. However, it is completely good to choose occupations that pay well but do not normally demand you to work more than 40 hours per week such as artist, writer, librarian, personal trainer, chiropractor, nutritionist etc. Not all stress is negative, especially when it stimulates you, keeps you active, makes you feel useful, and most significantly, generates some revenue.

2. Attempt remote jobs

Women who would require aid with mobility or would prefer working from home can attempt online employment and yet be able to produce money to fend for themselves without necessarily being dependent on the support of a provider.

These occupations also allow you to work at your own speed and regulate your workplace temperature. You would not have to bother wiping that perspiration in a conference meeting with your bosses or getting that little sleep to feel refreshed. The intriguing aspect is that some of these occupations demand little or no qualification in a certain sector, while you might potentially master others through experience and learning on the job. A classic example is the occupation linked with customer support. Some additional remote occupations include marketing coordinator, operations manager, patient care assistant (mother-baby), copywriter, etc. However, a large selection of these employment alternatives might be identified in just one or two searches on the internet to meet your desires. A handful of these vocations pay similarly well.

How can you stay healthy in your menopausal stage?
1. Stay consistent with your exercises.
One proven approach to maintaining a robust and active body is exercise. It might not necessarily imply that you have to go to the gym virtually every day or lift those hefty metals while gnashing your teeth, but playing those indoor games and being regular with your home exercises go a long way to aid with easy blood flow and discomfort in the joints. You may take a stroll while listening to your favorite song or speech or run a couple of times around the complex with your little ones. Swimming would undoubtedly deal with those heat flushes, even when you desire to exercise. These workouts not only benefit you physiologically but also protect you from too much pondering and boredom.
2. Regular health check-ups and take your medications as prescribed
It is usual to take those prescription drugs during your menopausal period as your body suffers hormonal fluctuations and other changes. It is vital to additionally visit the local health center as often as feasible to take your Follicle Stimulating Hormone (FSH) level checks, blood tests or urine tests, mammography, colonoscopy, lipid screening, bone density testing, etc. You might also attempt a home test by obtaining a self-test kit for women from drugstore outlets.
3. Prioritize self-care: This is a moment when you may need to focus on your physical and mental well-being more than ever. Prioritize getting enough sleep, exercising frequently, eating nutrient-dense meals, and drinking at least 8 glasses of water a day. to maintain your body and mind in peak form.
4. Cultivate meaningful relationships: Surround yourself with pleasant and encouraging individuals who will enrich your life. This might include family and friends or joining social groups or clubs that share your interests.

5. Pursue new interests: Menopause might be a terrific opportunity to pursue new hobbies or interests that you never had time for previously. This might involve learning a new language, practicing a new activity, or taking up a creative hobby like painting or writing.
6. Practice mindfulness. Menopause may be a time of transformation and transition. Mindfulness techniques like meditation or yoga can help you stay grounded and present, lowering stress and boosting general well-being.

CONCLUSION.

For too long, women have had to battle to understand the truth about menopause and to take up arms for their health and their sanity. Speaking up about the worries of a female body as it matures should be considered natural, not daring. Menopause isn't a death sentence. We must break with the sexist assumption that a woman's worth is related to her estrogen and her age. Instead, we could conceive of menopause as a new phase of life and the final period as merely one marker along the route. When women need support navigating their symptoms and the health consequences of menopause, clear, non-sexist information and proven remedies should be provided.

These changes are compounded by the effects of age, social and metabolic factors, daily activity, and well-being. Age at menopause reflects the complex interconnections of health and socioeconomic factors such as ethnicity, food, education, oral contraceptive use, weight, employment, exposure to endocrine-disrupting chemicals, alcohol consumption, smoking, and physical activity. Although menopause is normal, in certain situations ovarian failure can occur sooner than typical; this is pathological and necessitates rigorous biochemical studies to separate it from illnesses causing infertility. A variety of clinical issues affect elderly women, including endocrine, cardiovascular, skeletal, urogenital tract, and immunological systems; body mass; vasomotor tone; mood; and sleep pattern.

Maintaining physical activity and exercise during menopause can help alleviate some of the effects on strength. Strength training, including resistance exercises and weight-bearing activities, can help maintain muscle mass and bone density, which can help retain strength. Additionally, a good diet, proper sleep, and stress management skills can also assist in maintaining general strength and fitness throughout menopause.

Finally, in every stage of life, you are in the right position to define it. Ignore the cultural critics, be well-informed, and take charge of your menopausal age without looking back.